The Children's Hair Care Manual

A Step By Step Guide For Taking Care Of Your Child's Hair

AUTHOR BREANNA RUTTER

TABLE OF CONTENTS

INTRODUCTION TO
THE CHILDREN'S HAIR CARE MANUAL

"The Children's Hair Care Manual is a pocket guide that will help you to successfully take care of your child's hair. You may have chosen to pursue this self-education about children hair care for a variety of reasons; a curiosity to learn proper hair care or maybe because you have limited access to professional hair care services. Learning how to take care of your child's hair will take patience and cooperation from both you and your child/children. Kids have a hard time being patient and this manual will teach you tips on how to get their hair done in little time without much fuss. Dealing with temper tantrums can be the worst and you will learn how to avoid them by implementing tricks that will allow you to style and take care of their hair without them feeling uncomfortable during the process.

Taking care of your child's hair will take commitment from you no matter how busy or difficult life becomes because if you do not take care of your child's hair, it will become unhealthy from neglect. This manual will offer a variety of hairstyling options that you can allow for your child/children to wear that is both age appropriate and very simple to do. The most crucial part of this manual is the commitment of implementing an easy and simple to follow hair care regimen that has to be performed weekly.

Working with children's hair can be daunting but after reading this manual, you will know exactly what to do and what will work for your child's hair, I promise!

Please enjoy this informative read and have fun taking care of your child's hair during the process!" -Sincerely Breanna

1 HAIR CARE TOOLS

The tools used to take care of your child or children hair are extremely important when you are trying to maintain the health of their hair! There are a wide variety of hair care tools available on the market so don't allow yourself to become overwhelmed by their visual appeal. The most important thing to keep in mind when acquiring your hair care tools, is that they are constructed in a manner that does not compromise the health of your child's hair. New tools will always circulate and even if some actually gain popularity, there is no need to sway from your tools of choice if they meets your desired hair care needs.

The only hair tool that is necessary for detangling, maintaining, and grooming your child's hair is a seamless wide tooth detangling comb! This has always been the #1 secret to easy detangling no matter how fine, thick, course, silky, curly, straight, or wavy your child's hair is, you will always need a wide tooth comb for their detangling & grooming needs! This tool will prevent a great deal of tears and hard times when doing your child's hair, trust me!

What's just as important as a seamless wide tooth detangling comb are a pair of hair cutting shears. The beauty about children's hair is that is usually does not undergo much manipulation (such as wearing weaves, extensions, and using heat) when styling so trimming the ends of their hair will be done infrequently! Later on, we will discuss the importance of trimming your child's hair to keep it healthy and thriving. Refer to the chart on the following page to know the difference between safe and harsh hair care tools.

SAFE HAIR CARE TOOLS	HARSH HAIR CARE TOOLS
Seamless Wide Tooth Comb	Combs with Seams In-between the Teeth
Soft Boar Bristle Hair Brush	Plastic Bristle Hair Brush
Hair Cutting Shears (only to be used on hair)	Safety Scissors (Household Scissors)
Silk Hair Accessories	Cotton/Wool Hair Accessories
Ouch less/Seamless Hair Bands	Metal Bind/Plastic Bind On Hair Bands
Paddle Brush	Metal Wig Brush
Heat Styling Up To 350°	Heat Styling Over 350°
Blow Drying on Low-Medium Heat	Blow Drying on High Heat

2 DETANGLE

Properly detangling your child's hair is your first line of defense when protecting their hair from breakage and damage and also when protecting yourself from a temper tantrum! Use extreme gentleness when detangling their hair because children are less forgiving to snags from the comb and that is understandable if it is causing pain.

When you encounter a tangle, do not tug through it! Instead, remove the comb and free the tangle from the bottom, not the top, to make the entire process more gentler. Also every time you are detangling your child's hair, make sure to hold their hair with your other hand so that they do not feel any pain from their hair being handled. Sometimes just raking your fingers gently through their hair is enough for detangling and this usually works best if their hair is of a loose curly hair types but in most cases, a wide tooth comb is preferred. Also when detangling your child's hair, detangle infrequently to minimize the how often you handle their hair. It is best to only detangle your child's hair prior to shampoo washing, before a hair treatment, or before styling. Also, style your child's hair in a style that will last until their next shampoo or conditioner wash to limit detangling even more!

I will walk you step by step through how to detangle your child's hair properly no matter their texture or curl pattern!

Children Hair Detangle Regimen

Step #1 Generously apply a rinse conditioner to hair and wait a couple of minutes until hair has softened. Work in manageable sections (6-8 sections) from the tips to roots with a seamless wide tooth comb.

Do not apply product to the scalp as this causes buildup!

The last detangling stroke is when you can successfully comb once with ease through your section of hair!

Step #2 Loosely braid or twist each section after detangling and rinse out all traces of conditioner with warm water.

Step #3 With sections still loosely braided/twisted, final rinse with the coolest water they can stand to close cuticles for smooth frizz free hair.

Step #4 Pat towel dry, unravel sections and follow up with your hair treatment of choice or proceed to style working section by section!

3 SHAMPOO

When shampooing your child's hair, understand that a little shampoo goes a long way! In fact, black hair does not have to be shampooed as often as other hair types and because of this, there is the added pressure of finding the perfect shampoo that will not strip your child's hair of vital moisture. Commercial shampoos are usually filled with very stripping cleansing agents that often leave hair very dry after shampooing. Using a mild shampoo is all around better for preserving the health of hair because of its mild cleansing power. Additionally, every time you shampoo wash your child's hair, it is highly advisable that you perform a Deep Condition Treatment afterwords but if the shampoo does not cause a squeaky clean finish, skipping a Deep Conditioning Treatment is just fine!

A good guide for knowing how often to shampoo wash your children hair is at least once a week or once every two weeks. This will vary depending on how often you use hair products on your child's hair and the condition of their scalp and hair. If your child is into sports or generally a very active, do not shampoo their hair more than once a week. Instead, conditioner wash in the middle of the week and shampoo wash at the end of the week. Only shampoo wash according to their unique needs (which would be best) by paying attention to notice buildup of hair products, dandruff, odor, or complaints of an itchy scalp. Any or all of the above are good indicators that it would be a good time to shampoo wash your child's hair.

I will walk you step by step through how to shampoo your children hair and if you are in need of a quality shampoo, I highly suggest HowToBlackHair.com referred hair care products specifically formulated for maintaining healthy hair.

Children Hair Shampoo Regimen

Step #1 Follow the Children Hair Detangle Regimen.

Step #2 Apply shampoo directly to the scalp and message with finger pads to form a lather.

Step #3 Unravel a section and use lather to cleanse the ends then lightly re-braid or re-twist the section.

Repeat this step on all sections, one at a time.

Step #4 Rinse all traces of shampoo from hair with warm water.

Step #5 With sections still loosely braided/twisted, final rinse with the coolest water they can stand to close cuticles for smooth frizz free hair.

Step #6 Pat towel dry, unravel sections and follow up with your hair treatment of choice or proceed to style working section by section!

4 DEEP CONDITION

Children may need their hair deep conditioned from time to time to keep it healthy, especially if your child hair has problems with dryness! One of the reasons why many parents have to deep condition their child's hair more often is because it can be difficult to keep their hair protected during the night. Children can be pretty wild sleepers and this can cause their bonnet or head scarf to slip off during the night, leading to dry hair with every toss and turn!

Using a quality deep conditioning product will not be done frequently but, it is vital for incorporating much needed moisture into your child's hair. You will usually notice that during the hotter & drier times of year, more deep conditioning is required to quench their dry hair!

It is suggested to deep condition your children hair at least every two weeks. Deep conditioning their hair will vary sometimes depending on how tight their curl pattern is, your hair care styling habits, & usage of other hair products you use on your child's hair as well. Also, while deep conditioning their hair, remember to avoid adding product to their scalp as this causes buildup which leads to flaking and itchiness during the week!

Next, I will walk you step by step through how to deep condition your children hair properly from start to finish! If you are in need of a quality deep conditioner for your child's hair, I highly suggest HowToBlackHair.com referred hair care products specifically formulated for maintaining healthy hair.

Children Hair Deep Condition Regimen

Step #1 Begin with already detangled hair or allow the deep conditioner to help you detangle working on small sections at a time (6 to 8 sections).

Do not apply product to the scalp as this causes buildup!

Step #2 Saturate the ends first with deep conditioner & loosely rebraid or retwist each section.

Deep condition as suggested by the product or cover your hair with a shower cap and process for 30 minutes max.

Step #3 While sections are still loosely braided or twisted, thoroughly rinse all traces of deep conditioner from hair with warm water.

Step #4 Final rinse with the coolest water they can stand to close cuticles for smooth frizz free hair.

Step #5 Pat towel dry, unravel your sections, and proceed to follow up with your styling of choice!

5 CONDITIONER WASH

One of the best ways to keep your child's hair healthy especially for pleasing chronically dry hair is to co wash (conditioner wash) to re-moisturize their hair to a great extent! Healthy hair is kept moisturized which will prevent it from becoming dry and breaking! The key to any successful hair care regimen has always been an incorporation of co-washing.

Co-wash means to wash your hair with conditioner alone and this is a great way to re-moisturize and also cleanse your child's hair for the time being, instead of shampoo washing frequently. It is preferred to use an inexpensive water based conditioning product to serve as your child's co-wash conditioner so that it can also aid you with detangling. Rinse Conditioners/Co Wash Conditioners are usually used frequently and in large quantities so having an adequate supply of this conditioner is important when helping you maintain the health of child's hair.

A good guide for knowing how often to conditioner wash children hair is at least twice a week or weekly. The frequency of co washing your child's will depend on how well their hair can retain moisture. Tighter curl patterns (like Type 4 Hair) often need more moisturizing care than a looser curl pattern (like Type 3 Hair). You can of course only co wash according to their unique needs (which would be best) by paying attention to notice if their hair feels dry. Co-washing is also a way to cleanse hair when needed, but co-washing cannot replace a much needed shampoo wash!

I will walk you step by step through how to co-wash your child's hair and if you are in need of a quality conditioner, I suggest HowToBlackHair.com referred hair care products specifically formulated for maintaining healthy hair.

Children Hair Conditioner Wash Regimen

Step #1 Generously apply a rinse conditioner to hair and wait a couple of minutes until hair has softened. Work in manageable sections (6-8 sections) from the tips to roots with a seamless wide tooth comb.

Do not apply product to the scalp as this causes buildup!

The last detangling stroke is when you can successfully comb once with ease through the section of hair!

Step #2 Loosely braid or twist each section after detangling and rinse out all traces of conditioner with warm water.

Step #3 With sections still loosely braided/twisted, final rinse with the coolest water they can stand to close cuticles for smooth frizz free hair.

Step #4 Pat towel dry, unravel sections and follow up with your hair treatment of choice or proceed to style working section by section!

6 PROTEIN LEAVE IN

Protein leave in products are better for children hair than protein treatments because kids are usually less tolerable when dealing with bad smells and being patient! This makes performing protein treatments difficult so instead, use a protein leave in when needed for your child. For your child's hair or anyone else's hair health, balancing elasticity keeps hair healthy! Protein strengthens weak, gummy and/or fine hair. Moisture (water/water based products) allows the hair to become more flexible and softer. If your child has natural hair, it usually does not require protein because it has not been stripped of its protein unlike chemically relaxed hair. Protein has to be used often on hair that is chemically relaxed because this hair lacks its naturally occurring protein. Applying protein unnecessarily to your child's hair will harden it! In regards to moisture, it's near impossible to over moisturize your child's hair unless you are giving them deep conditioning treatments more than once a week!

The frequency of using a protein leave in on your children hair depends on if they have relaxed or natural hair. On natural hair, usage once a week for fine hair is suggested and for course hair once every two weeks is suggested. For relaxed hair, no matter if your children have course or fine hair, its required to be used 2 times or 3 times a week. Using a little bit of protein leave in on your child's relaxed hair every other day is just fine but lessen up if you think their hair is becoming stiff, hard, or crunchy.

I will walk you step by step through how to use a protein leave in on your child's hair! If you are in need of a quality protein leave in, I highly suggest HowToBlackHair.com referred hair care products specifically formulated for maintaining healthy hair.

Children Hair Protein Leave In Regimen

Step #1 Begin with already clean detangled hair (it can be wet or dry).

Step #2 Lather a small amount of protein leave in in your hands and apply on the hair working on one manageable section at a time (6 to 8 sections of hair).

Do not apply product to the scalp as this causes buildup!

Step #3 Proceed to style your child's hair!

HAIR TIP: Working section by section, blow dry on warm to raise the cuticles (refer to definition guide), apply protein leave in and then blow dry on cool. This helps the protein product penetrate faster into your child's hair ultimately adding strength and balancing their hair elasticity!

7 LEAVE IN MOISTURIZER

The leave in moisturizer you will use for your children hair will add moisture into their hair on the whim without much fuss or wait usually from a deep conditioning process! It has been suggested according to the detangle regimen to detangle with a rinse conditioner/co-wash conditioner but if you want to detangle with a leave in moisturizer instead, that's an option as well. The reason why detangling with a leave in moisturizer was not suggested for the detangle regimen is because leave in moisturizers are designed to moisturize your hair internally while a rinse conditioner is designed to just attract water to the outer surface of hair, which aids you best when detangling your child's hair.

A good guide for knowing how often to apply a leave in moisturizer to your children hair is bi-weekly or weekly. The frequency of applying a leave in moisturizer to their hair will vary depending on how tight their curl pattern is and how well their hair can retain moisture. Tighter curl patterns (like Type 4 Hair) often need more moisturizing attention than a looser curl pattern (like Type 3 Hair). With this product, you have to experiment applying it on damp or dry hair to find out when applying it to your child's hair is best. Many parents prefer applying a leave in on almost dry hair because children don't usually have the temperament to sit through getting their hair done while water drips down their neck and face! Leave a dry towel wrapped around their head until their hair is almost dry before applying the leave in moisturizer.

I will walk you step by step through how to moisturize your children hair and if you are in need of a quality leave in moisturizer, I highly suggest HowToBlackHair.com referred hair care products specifically formulated for maintaining healthy hair.

Children Hair Leave In Moisturizer Regimen

Step #1 Follow the Child Hair Detangle Regimen but allow hair to air dry while in sections with an absorbent towel wrapped around their head.

Step #2 With hair almost dry or at least damp without dripping, apply leave in moisturizer to hair section by section.

Do not apply product to the scalp as this causes buildup!

Step #3 For increased moisture (if you struggle with maintaining dry hair) incorporate the LOC Method (refer to the definition guide)

Step #4 Proceed to style working on one section at a time.

If you like to style dried hair, allow hair to air dry or blow dry preferably with low heat.

8 OIL SEALANT

An oil sealant will limit the amount of times you need to re-moisturize your child's hair. Do not skip applying an oil sealant to your children hair so that your moisturizing efforts aren't becoming a waste of time. The purpose of using an oil sealant in their hair care regimen, is to slow down the rate of water evaporating from their strands of hair. To clarify, there is no such thing as a permanent sealant that will keep your child's hair moisturized forever because a sealant like that will most likely damage their hair, prevent you from effectively using heat, and make chemical treatments like deep conditioning and relaxing ineffective. Keep in mind that the heavier or thicker your oil sealant of choice is, the longer their hair can retain moisture and also the more greasy their hair will feel depending on their texture of hair. Learn more about how the texture of hair determines what hair care practices and products are best by referring to The Natural Hair Bible or The Relaxed Hair Bible!

An oil sealant is to be used before or after applying your leave in moisturizer. If you adopt the LOC Method, sealing your hair with oil will be done before your creamy leave in moisturizer is applied to your hair. Depending on your child's hair, oils like Coconut oil would be great or heavier oils/butters like Castor oil or Shea Butter can work depending on their grade of hair. For the majority, tighter curl patterns lean more towards heavier oils/butters and looser curl patterns, lean more towards lighter oils.

I will walk you step by step through how to oil seal your child's hair and if you are in need of a quality oil sealant, I highly suggest HowToBlackHair.com referred hair care products specifically formulated for maintaining healthy hair.

Children Hair Oil Sealant Regimen

Step #1 (Without the LOC Method)

Lightly coat fingers with your oil/butter of choice and lubricate damp hair or almost dry hair in manageable sections at a time

Oil seal preferably AFTER applying your creamy leave in moisturizer, or Oil seal on damp product free hair

Focus on the ends of your hair as this needs the most coverage when maintaining moisturized hair!

Step #2 (With the LOC Method for Constant Dry Hair)

Lightly coat fingers with your oil/butter or choice and lubricate manageable sections at a time RIGHT BEFORE applying your creamy leave in moisturizer

After applying your oil, apply your creamy leave in moisturizer to complete the LOC Method

Step #3 After sections are sealed, proceed to style working on one section at a time. If you like to style dried hair, allow hair to air dry or blow dry preferably with low heat

9 HAIR CARE REGIMEN

I have explained the purpose of each hair care product that you will need to take care of your child's hair, how often to apply them and more importantly, directions on how to apply them! The children hair care regimen will allow you to take great care of your child's hair because you will be equipped with an easy guide that you can follow weekly to help you maintain their hair. As you may have observed, taking care of your child's hair has to always be done in sections being that there is a preferred way to handle hair to avoid pain while combing and styling. Understanding how to do a variety of simple hair care techniques all contribute to their overall hair care regimen.

So of course it's almost a given that you still do not understand how to implement a regimen that will work for you because each product regimen can make you feel overwhelmed as well as leave you to assume that you have to handle your hair frequently, which is quite the opposite.

Follow along with the suggested weekly hair care regimen that will be explained next and keep in mind that the chart is 100% flexible to your child's unique hair care needs. One week you may feel the need to tweak certain parts of the hair care regimen so feel free to make changes that are necessary for your child.

I will walk you step by step through an awesome hair care regimen that you can use as a guide for taking care of your child's hair and in the following sections, we will discuss various hairstyling options.

Children Hair Care Regimen	
(WEEK 1/DAY 1) *Detangle(mandatory) *Shampoo(mandatory) *Deep Condition (mandatory) *Leave In Moisturizer (mandatory) *Oil Sealant (mandatory)	(WEEK 2/DAY 1) *Detangle(mandatory) *Shampoo(mandatory) *Leave In Moisturizer (mandatory) *Oil Sealant (mandatory)
(WEEK 1/DAY 2)	(WEEK 2/DAY 2)
(WEEK 1/DAY 3)	(WEEK 2/DAY 3)
(WEEK 1/DAY 4) *Conditioner Wash(optional) *Leave In Moisturizer or Protein Leave In (optional) *Oil Sealant (optional)	(WEEK 2/DAY 4) *Conditioner Wash(optional) * Leave In Moisturizer or Protein Leave In (optional) *Oil Sealant (optional)
(WEEK 1/DAY 5)	(WEEK 2/DAY 5)
(WEEK 1/DAY 6)	(WEEK 2/DAY 6)
(WEEK 1/DAY 7) *Conditioner Wash(optional) * Leave In Moisturizer or Protein Leave In (optional) *Oil Sealant (optional)	(WEEK 1/DAY 7) *Conditioner Wash(optional) * Leave In Moisturizer or Protein Leave In (optional) *Oil Sealant (optional)
Continue to repeat this 2 WEEK Cycle	

10 HAIRSTYLING OPTIONS

Opposite to what many people may think, children can sport a variety of hairstyles that look beautiful as well as complimentary to their age and level of maturity. The key to picking the best styles for your children hair depends on how well they can handle styles whether it be braids, twists or while free. Small children don't do well with maintaining free hair, like a twist out or braid out, because they will often get food or dirt in their hair and cause tangles from touching it. Those styles would only be fitting for children who can keep their hands out of their hair and even better, retwist their own hair at night to maintain their look! There are so many ways to make hairstyling work for you and your child, it just takes a little bit of hairstyling skills on your part. For detailed step by step instructions on styling hair in a variety of hairstyles, check out HowToBlackHair.com!

Before I begin to teach and offer you some hairstyling choices for your child's hair, I will first address the concern about children wearing weaves and extensions. Many parents have an issue with children wearing weaves, extensions and even relaxing their hair and this debate will never end because everyone has their idea of what hairstyles are proper for a child and not. The problems with treating your child's hair in those ways is that it easily becomes a crutch for busy parents and sometimes, the child's hair is just too fragile to handle additional hair. I have personally witnessed many parents leaving installs in their child's hair for months at a time and then when it comes to removing them, they just remove the weave, shampoo and install another weave! The health of your child's hair rests in your hands! I am not against installs for children, but I do encourage safer styles for children that allow their hair to flourish as well as encourage you to care for their hair best without restrictions!

Children Hairstyling Options

TWIST OUT OR BRAID OUT

Take small to medium sized sections of damp or dry moisturized hair and twist clockwise or counter clockwise. For braid outs, braid over hand and underhand alternately. Alternating your direction per braid or twist allows the most volume and will avoid clumping! After hair dries (pinch to check for wetness) unravel twists or braids for the completed look! If you separate the braid out or twist out further for fullness, you will have to reset the hairstyle sooner!

MINI TWISTS

Preferably begin with small to medium sized sections of damp moisturized hair and twist in any direction you choose. Once dry, the style is complete! During the week, unravel the twists to sport a twist out.

STRAW ROD SET

Take a small to medium sized section of damp moisturized hair and smooth fingers down the section to locate the ends. Wrap the bottom most part around the straw two to three times and then roll the section around the surface of the straw. Tuck the top of the straw downwards and use a rubber band or a closed bobby pin to secure the fold. Once dry, unloose the secure and unravel straw in the opposite direction to give no resistance to the new formed curls! During the week, unravel each individual spiral to sport a bigger fluffier look! For more hairstyling options, visit our hair care & styling website at HowToBlackHair.com!

11 NIGHT TIME ROUTINE

Your child's night time routine is vital for preserving the health of their hair and without this routine, they will constantly suffer from breakage and you will have to restyle throughout the week! Not only does handling your children hair in a gentle manner dramatically decrease breakage, but so does your protective night time routine!

When performing the night time routine, it is very important that their hair is re-twisted, re-braided, bunned, or pineappled (refer to the definition guide) to preserve the look of their hairstyle. Before going to bed, always protect their hair with appropriate material to eliminate friction encountered throughout the night. The two choices of fabric that are best for protecting your children hair while sleeping are Satin and Silk.

Satin is more affordable than silk, is the more flexible material and can be washed with ease. Satin does not cause friction on hair or edges nor does Silk, but Satin causes more friction in comparison to Silk.

Silk is priced higher than satin, is not as flexible in comparison and has to be delicately hand washed or cleansed through a dry cleaning service. Silk does not cause friction on hair or edges and nor does Satin, but Silk is superior in preventing friction than Satin.

For children, it is preferred to protect their hair during the night with a Satin or Silk bonnet or pillowcase. Using a Satin or Silk headscarf can slip throughout the night ruining your protective efforts!

NIGHT TIME ROUTINE

Step #1 (For Satin/Silk Bonnet)

Wear a comfortable but secure bonnet that covers all of your child's hair If the bonnet feels tight or too loose to stay secure, seek another bonnet or protection of choice.

Step #2 (For Satin/Silk Pillowcase)

Cover your bed pillow of choice with your case of choice. Double case your pillow if needed because of slippage.

12 TRIMMING HAIR ENDS

Trimming the ends of your child's hair does not mean give them a haircut! The difference between a trim and a haircut is the amount of hair you choose to remove of course but this does not stop many individuals from mistakenly trimming off too much hair. To know if your child truly needs a trim is by taking notice to see a consistent thickness of hair near the ends. If the ends look thin, it's time for a trim and an even better way is to observe if there is visible damage on the ends of their hair. If you never get your children hair ends dusted or trimmed, it will lead to chronic breakage and dryness which leads to unhealthy hair that constantly shortens in length! Refer to The Natural Hair Bible or The Relaxed Hair Bible to understand the importance of trimming the ends of your hair and what the author suffered through after two years of never trimming!

Trimming or dusting the ends of your children hair should be no more than 1/2 an inch if you keep their ends in good health. If the ends of their hair are severely damaged, it is highly suggested that you seek a professional cut to ensure that the damage is trimmed of appropriately.

I will walk you step by step through how to trim or dust the ends of your child hair if you do wish to do it on your own but if you are not 100% comfortable with cutting your child's hair, seek a professional in your area to do this!

Children Hair Trimming Ends

ONLY USE CUTTING SHEARS EXCLUSIVELY
USED FOR TRIMMING YOUR HAIR!

(TRIMMING DAMAGED ENDS W/ CURLY HAIR)

Step #1 Begin with damp detangled hair and position your child in a well lit room with plenty of light to assist you.

Step #2 Starting in the back of the head, part a horizontal line of hair at the nape of the neck and use gator clips/duck bill clips to keep the rest of your hair sectioned out of the way. Always work in small sections at a time!

Step #3 Take a small section of detangled hair, twist to the ends, and trim about an 1/8 inch of hair to dust for maintenance. Your child's dusted hair ends should look like little flecks of hair. For a trim that requires more than an 1/8 of length lost, consult with a professional to aid you so that you don't accidently perform an uneven trim!

(TRIMMING DAMAGED ENDS W/ RELAXED HAIR)

Step #1 Begin with dry detangled hair and position yourself in a well lit room with plenty of light to assist you

Step #2 Follow Step 2 & Step 3 from above carefully

AFTERWORDS

"This manual was created in mind for parents who want to take care of their children's hair in the best way they possibly can! That of course begins with educating yourself about the basic needs of your child's hair, how to use a variety of hair care products as well to preserve the health of their hair along the way. You may have chosen to read this guide because you support my work, you were looking for information on children hair care, or you were looking for this information to help a loved one. As a child I don't remember having an actual hair care regimen but I do remember getting my hair relaxed faithfully every 3 weeks or month. That is not best practice when relaxing a child's hair let alone anyone's hair but with limited access to funds and hair care knowledge, my hair care was left up to my mother and I. As I have gotten older, I learned so much along the way realizing that a lot of things I was using on my hair and doing to my hair at a young age was the detriment to my stagnant length and persistent scalp eczema. For my own reasons as expressed in my book., The Relaxed Hair Bible, I no longer relax my hair and being natural, I have seen my hair flourish in health and length better than I have ever experienced with my hair.

It is important that you follow the recommended hair care regimen equipped with quality hair care products that you and your child can benefit from as you continue to take care of their hair.

I hope that you thoroughly enjoyed this read because it was a pleasure of mine to write this for your knowledge and enjoyment!"

Sincerely, Breanna

ADDITIONAL RESOURCES

The Official Website: www.Howtoblackhair.com

The Online Store: www.HowtoblackhairStore.com

Free Subscription Email: http://eepurl.com/FZs5b

For Additional Hair Questions

YourHairQuestions@Gmail.com

Black Hair Styling Tutorials

BlackWomenHair YouTube Channel

www.Youtube.com/BlackWomenHair

HowToBlackHair YouTube Channel

www.Youtube.com/HowToBlackHair

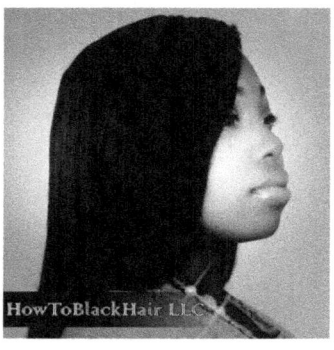

The Natural Hair Bible

The 10 Commandments of Black Hair Care

www.HowToBlackHair.com

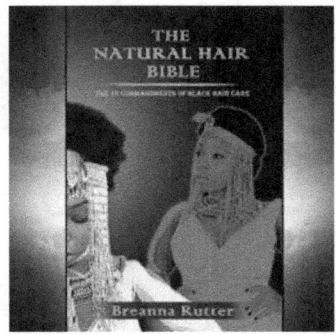

The Relaxed Hair Bible

The 10 Commandments of Long Healthy Relaxed Hair

www.HowToBlackHair.com

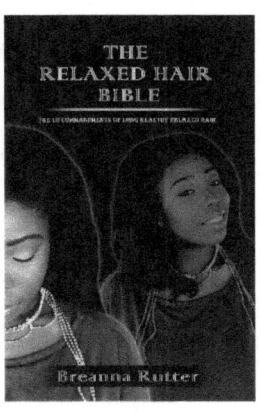

Black Hair Styling DVDs (Over 20+ Hairstyles)

www.HowToBlackHair.com

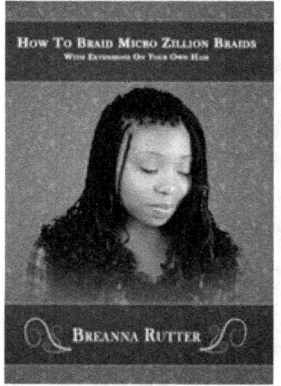

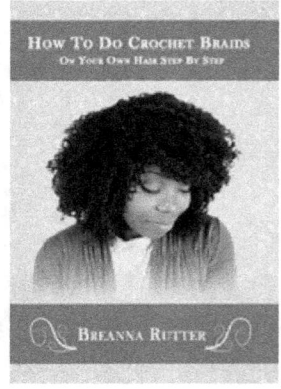

DEFINITION GUIDE

Curl Pattern: *the natural curl pattern of your hair strands according to the LOIS or Andre Walker hair typing system*
Cuticles: *a naturally protecting shield (arranged like shingles to the roof of a home) outside of your hair strands*
Dusting: *trimming about an 1/8 inch of hair from the ends*
Elasticity: *the stretching ability of your hair*
LOC Method: *layering products for moisture in the order of; Liquid (leave in moisturizer or water), Oil, Cream (thick consistency moisturizer/sealant like a hair butter)*
Pineapple: *putting hair in a high bun or ponytail for bed time to avoid smashed curls and preserve a style that consists of free hair*
Texture: *the feel and absorbency of your hair based on the LOIS Hair Typing System*

INDEX

HOW TO BLACK HAIR LLC.
WRITTEN BY BREANNA RUTTER
BOOK DESIGNED BY BREANNA RUTTER
COVER DESIGNED BY JARED RUTTER
ALL RIGHTS RESERVED.
VISIT WWW.HOWTOBLACKHAIR.COM

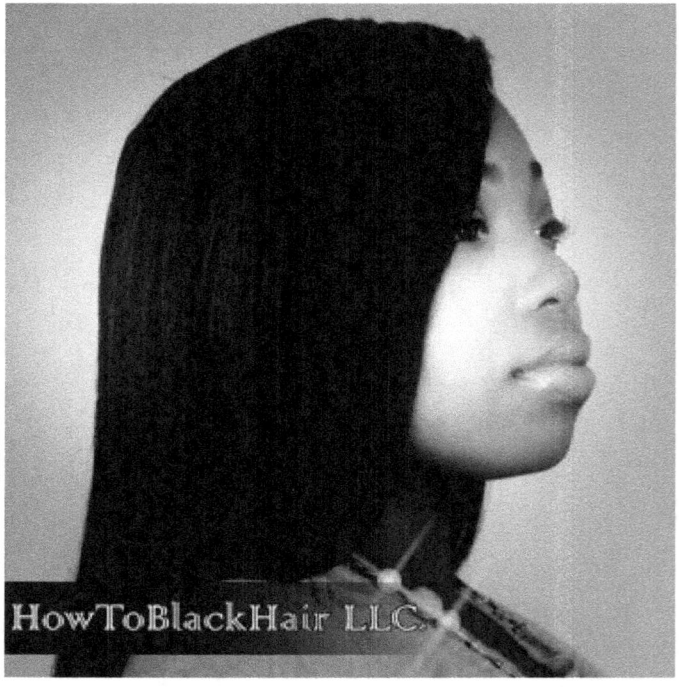